Fighting Alzheimer's Disease

Major Steps To Maintain
Cognitive Skills and Wellness

Fighting Alzheimer's Disease

Major Steps To Maintain
Cognitive Skills and Wellness

TERENCE McCARTHY

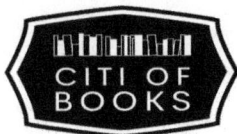

CITI OF
BOOKS

CITIOFBOOKS, INC.
3736 Eubank NE Suite A1
Albuquerque, NM 87111-3579
www.citiofbooks.com
Hotline: 1 (877) 389-2759
Fax: 1 (505) 930-7244

Ordering Information:
Quantity sales. Special discounts are available on quantity purchases by corporations, associations, and others. For details, contact the publisher at the address above.

Printed in the United States of America.
ISBN-13:   Softcover   978-1-959682-19-6
                    eBook   978-1-959682-20-2

Library of Congress Control Number: 2022919778

Foreword

This book is a WAKE UP CALL for all persons 60 and over and for those under 60 who are experiencing Mild Cognitive Impairment (MCI). With all of us living longer and surviving medical maladies that previously terminated many lives, the threat of Alzheimer's disease (AD) is now looming larger than life with approximately 5.3 million persons in the United States probably diagnosed with AD. I use the qualifier "probably" because no one to date has been conclusively diagnosed with AD until after death by an autopsy. Currently in this year -2016 - the chances of someone coming down with AD are: 13% for persons over 65 and 50% for persons over 85. If someone over 60 chooses not to pro-actively respond to this challenge, he or she is carelessly risking to be overtaken by AD and at the same time, is unnecessarily subjecting his or her loved ones to 2 to 20 years of a 24/7 burden of care giving.

Prologue

The author has spent the last five years studying medical journals including the 483 page comprehensive book on Alzheimer's disease (AD) published by the Mayo Clinic in 2013. Other research and studies mainly consisted of snapshot reports of different aspects of strategies and measures which individuals could use to delay the onset of AD. No concise, methodical compilation of this data has appeared in print.

After spending the last 32 years in ministering to people in a hospital and an assisted living facility, the author who is now 81, has been exposed to many persons with onset AD and is completely aware that AD is terminal and has no cure. This intimate experience with many AD victims and the fact that the author's research has revealed that no single brief document exists to guide persons over the age of 60 in developing effective strategies and measures to delay the onset of AD, has led the author to putting this comprehensive guide together.

Considering the probable exponential increase in AD cases from the current level of 5.3 Americans to a projected 10 million by 2025, there is a critical need to educate more people over 60 about this enormous and deadly threat and to get them performing in a more pro-active and effective manner to delay the seemingly inevitable onset of Alzheimer's disease.

Section I

General

Curing Alzheimer's disease (AD) is not currently achievable. However, there are several steps that show promise collectively deterring AD.

AD is the most common cause of dementia among adults age 65 and older. AD is a neurodegenerative disease in which cognition becomes more impaired as the brain's nerve cells degenerate and communication pathways break down.

The course AD may take is variable. It may last from 2 to 20 years afrer first symptoms appear. As things stand right now, the disease once diagnosed is terminal.

There are two types of AD:
-        Early onset - before age 60.

-        Typical AD - at age 60 or older.

Some of the earliest signs and symptoms of dementia due to Alzheimer's disease include:

- Memory loss

- Difficulty in performing familiar tasks Problems with language, for example: misnaming objects or inability to find an appropriate word in conversations

- Disorientation in time or place

- Poor judgement

- Problems with calculating numbers

- Misplacing/losing personal items

- Mood swings

- Personality changes

- Losing initiative

AD affects the brain by destroying its most basic components -especially the nerve cells (neurons) that relay messages within the brain and between the brain and the rest of the body.

Gradually, the disease prevents people from performing routine self-care and doing household tasks that they have performed for many years. As AD spreads through the brain and more nerve cells die, the size of the brain shrinks. This change can be detected in brain imaging.

Two abnormal structures in the brain are the cause of AD - amyloid plaques and neurofibrillary tangles.

Plaques are large indissoluble clumps found between and around living nerve cells. These plaques consist mainly of a protein called amyloid-beta. The amyloid-beta dumps are protein fragments cut off by enzymes from the amyloid precursor protein. The amyloid-beta fragments tend to stick together forming hardened dumps of plaques. The role of the amyloid-beta dumps is not clearly known since some people are more resistant to damage from amyloid-beta than others, thus, enabling them to live longer without noticeable cognitive impairments.

Neurofibrillary tangles are the other characteristic structure of AD. Tangles occur inside a cell body and are caused by the breakdown of a protein called tau. As AD develops, the tau portions undergo chemical changes causing it to malfunction. Strands of tau unravel and clump together forming tangled masses. This produces a devastating effect on a neuron causing disruption in the transportation of nucrient and electronic impulses within the cell body. This leads to a breakdown of vital cell functions. Studies indicate that tau is key to how toxic amyloid beta is to neurons.

Although amyloid-beta plaques and tangles are prominent features of AD, there are several other factors that can play a part in the disease process. These are: genetic mutations, vascular brain injury, type 2 diabetes and chronic high blood pressure.

Overall, more research is required to provide a more precise picture of what specific causes are indeed responsible for the development of AD.

Section 2

The Development of Strategies to Deter the Risk of Developing Alzheimer's Disease (AD)

Various studies indicate that strategies such as staying mentally sharp and developing life style habits may reduce the risk of developing Alzheimer's disease - these include exercising, eating a diet rich in fruits and vegetables, participating in mentally stimulating activities and staying socially connected. All of the above should be engaged in by persons who are 60 or over. To set the stage for the consideration of these strategies, these points are presented.

Effect of Aging. The following changes in brain function naturally occur:

- It takes one longer to learn new things

- It can be harder to recall facts such as names, dates and places

- It becomes more difficult to handle more than one task at a time

- There are memory lapses such as where one keeps car keys or where one parked a car.

Points that usually remain unaffected by aging:

- Storage of language and word meanings
- Creativity
- Wisdom
- Procedural Memory- the storing of skills chat one has done repeatedly.

Strategy for improving everyday memory

- Keep a calendar

    ■ Helps prevent memory lapses and overcomes being overloaded with too many details

        • Establish this as a habit and it would be stored in procedural memory

        • Use a paper date book or a smart phone

        • Track information such as events, tasks, addresses or phone numbers

        • Designate separate sections in date book or smart phone

        • Regularly use the system

- Mark completed tasks.

- Organize clutter

  - Store frequently used items in same place -for keys, kitchen items and toolbox

  - Prioritize correspondence - required responses, information to consult and information for leisure.

- Focus Attention - slow down and focus on the present, look closely at person or tasks in front of you.

- Minimize distractions -turn radio, TV and cell phone off for 3 hours.

- Do one task at a time.

- Use selective attention - ignore surrounding noises.

- Use memory tricks - make associations, use related details.

- Employ other memory techniques - break it down, picture it, write it down, use cues such as notes.

- Brain aerobics -Involve a mental process that actively weighs and calculates different courses of action, consider activities such as mahjong titans, crosswords, sudoku, bridge and chess.

-     Vary routine.

-     Focus on speed by timing different events.

-     Try new things such as stay curious, volunteer at school or a charity, stay up to date on new technology, travel, stay socially active, attend local concerts and become active in church ministry.

-     Identify things you are doing right.

-     List behaviors that could use improvement.

-     Select one strategy you would like to work on first.

-     Lastly -

  •   Trust yourself instead saying" I cannot remember names.

  •   Move from blaming yourself to positive messages.

  •   Be patient with yourself

  •   Take one day at a time.

Developing A Healthy Life Style

There is no question that a healthy life style can control the development of Alzheimer's disease. The good news is the habits that have the greatest potential for reducing the risk of AD are also ones that may have the greatest impact on improving overall health and happiness.

The most important and effective life style factor is physical activity. Physical exertion increases blood flow to the brain which increases the supply of oxygen and nutrients to brain cells. This also tends to boost mood and energy levels which can sharpen mental processing and energy output. Exercise may also promote regeneration of brain cells and the development of new ones.

For the greatest benefits of physical exercise, one needs to look at the published findings of the federal government's Physical Activity Guidelines Committee which follows: First: Muscular Health. Two strength resistance training sessions per week will provide increases in strength and power and a recouping of lost muscle. Second: Bone Health. Four hours of aerobic exercise per week will provide an increase in bone mineral density and reduction in the risk of fracture. Third: Functional Health. Ninety minutes a week including aerobic and strength resistance training will provide almost 30 per cent reduction in age associated inability to carry out daily activities and result in reducing the risk of falls. Fourth: Meneal Health. Two and a half hours of aerobic and strength training exercises will result in the lowered risk of Alzheimer's disease.

Exercise Options

- Aerobic Exercise - Try to do aerobic exercises - this includes walking, running, cycling, stairclimbing and elliptical machines - five times a week. Start and finish with a slow pace. Be able to carry on a conversation during the exercise - chis will insure you are not overdoing it. Schedule the exercise on a calendar so that it won't be missed.

- Strength Resistance workouts - try to schedule these workouts two times a week but not on consecutive days. Seek a professional trainer to get the following advice: which 3 upper and 3 lower body exercises are best for you on exercise machines where the weights can be set. For example, sit at an abduction machine and initially set the weights at a maximum level. Reduce the weight by 15 pounds. Do two sets of 12 repetitions with a one minute break. Why is chis exercise so important?Studies have conclusively shown that a person loses muscle mass at the rate of 25% between the ages of 30 and 70 and 25% more between the ages of 70 and 90. The strength resistance exercises are designed so that one can completely recoup muscle mass loss. The great danger is that as one grows older, he or she is completely unaware of this massive muscle loss. <u>The result is that massive muscle loss makes a person highly vulnerable to losing</u>

<u>his/her balance, falling and breaking a hip bone.</u> A survey conducted in the US three years ago on persons over 55 who fell and broke a hip revealed the following data: Over 320,000 persons over 55 fell and broke their hips. Twenty-five per cent - 80,000 - died within 12 months; 50 % or 160,00 went into assisted living facilities and have yet to return home; and only 80,000 returned to independent life styles after 12 months.

Don't let any obstacle get in the way to participating five days each week in an exercise program. Please be assured that if anyone adopts any of the six obstacles listed below, he or she will be greatly increasing the risk for developing Alzheimer's disease. The six biggest obstacles are:

- 1. "I never have enough time".
- 2. 'I'm too old to start now".
- 3. "My health isn't good enough".
- 4. 'I'm too tired for exercise".
- 5. 'I'm not overweight, what's the point".
- 6. "It's too painful".

The other life style considerations are listed below:

- Eat Healthy - Studies support that food choices may help a brain function at its prime and significantly reduce the risk of developing AD. Recommend one consider the Mediterranean diet which focuses on fish, vegetables, fruits and olive oil. Avoid fried foods and make three days a week meatless.

- Sleep Well - A good night's sleep allows the body to rest and leaves one feeling refreshed the next day. Sufficient sleep - 7 to 9 hours - is extremely important for keeping the brain and the nervous system working properly. Sleep appears to have an impact on neurons, vital neuron connections, learning and memory processing. The following tips apply to getting quality sleep:

  o Try to go to bed at the same time each night.

  o Make it a habit to enjoy a quiet, soothing environment in the bedroom.

  o Remove distractions such as radios, TV and computers.

  o Get rid of bright lights and extraneous noises.

  o Avoid caffeine, nicotine, alcohol and late night meals.

- Drinking Alcohol - Drink alcohol in moderation.Men can have two 5 ounce drinks with dinner and women one 5 ounce drink. This practice will help to lower risks of AD.

- Drinking Water - One of the more serious aging problems is drinking sufficient water. The problem is due to the reduction of the body's thirst stimulus. This can cause significant dehydration which can be avoided by drinking 8 twelve ounce glasses of water on a daily basis which helps to reduce the risk of developing AD. Water is an essential element for a healthy brain and brain cells. Please note: A good indicator of dehydration status is to check the color of urine after strenuous exercise. Urine that is a dark yellow indicates that a serious dehydration exists. Drinking two to three 12 ounce glasses of water needs to be done immediately.

Section 3

Fighting Alzheimer's Disease

Once a person has been diagnosed with Alzheimer's disease (AD), most research has determined that it is too late to stop the neurodegenerative disorder or to reverse major neuron damage related to AD. So, the opportunity to fight onset AD is not a viable action.

However, reports in the summer of 2015 indicate that Australian scientists have found a way to reverse AD in 75% of mice they have treated. They have come up with a high speed ultrasound technology that clears mice brains of amyloid plaques. The ultrasound (focused therapeutic ultrasound) used is unique. It produces waves that oscillate super-fast and are able to stimulate the brains microglial cells to become active. The microglial cells are the waste removal cells in the brain. When they become stimulated, they can remove the amyloid plaques. Not only were the treated mice relieved of amyloid plaques, they demonstrated improved performance on memory tests. Where the mice had a complete removal of the amyloid plaques, researchers discovered a full restoration of memory. No side effects were noted and there was no damage detected in any of the surrounding brain tissue. There is hope that within the coming years - no date has been set - that persons with AD can be successfully treated. So the bottom line now is to do everything possible to slow down the development of AD since the potential exists to someday reverse AD.

The battle to fight AD is left to the mildly cognitive impaired under 60 and all individuals 60 and over - even in those situations where none is experiencing any cognitive impaired symptoms. The fighting of AD consists of the following measures and therapies including the Weekly Exercise Program in Section 4:

- The following vitamin supplement anti-oxidants are recommended:

  o Curcumin - This reduces systemic inflammation, relieves pain and more importantly crosses the blood-brain barrier. And then, it boosts cognitive functions and helps clear amyloid plaque. Curcumin can be found in Cosco under the label: Turmeric. It also can be found in CVS under the label: Turmeric.

  o Ubiquinol - This is a more bioavailable form of CoQlO. It is one of the most powerful fat-soluble anti-oxidants. Because ubiquinol is fat soluble, it can penetrate deep inside brain tissue and protect neurons from the ravages of oxidative stress damage. Ubiquinol can be found in Cosco under the label: Qunol Ubiquinol. It also can be found in CVS under the label: Qunol Ultra CoQlO.

- Hydrogen Water (H2) - Is an extraordinary anti-oxidant, a free radical destroyer that selectively ravenges the most dangerous and destructive hydroxyl radicals. H2 "nano" cells enter the mitochondria and cross the blood-brain barrier. The benefits of H2 therapy have been demonstrated in a wide range of conditions including Alzheimer's disease, vascular disease and diabetes. H2 is available via tablets of micronized elemental magnesium. To order go to ActiveH2.com. Under Purative Active H2 select: *www. drvitaminsoluble. com.*

- Mind-Set Meditation - Has been proven to lower high blood pressure and slash heart attacks by 50%. A review of 150 studies concluded that mind-set meditation has positive effects on stress, anxiety, depression, neuroses, degenerative diseases of aging (including AD), mental alertness and memory. The impact of chis technique when practiced 20 minutes in the morning and afternoon on a daily basis provides a significant reduction in the risks of developing Alzheimer's disease.

- Coffee - In addition to enhancing concentration, improving endurance and protecting against diabetes, epidemiologistical research suggests that moderate daily caffeinated coffee consumption helps reduce developing AD. Scientists discovered that people who drank three to five cups of coffee each day may reduce the risk of developing AD by as much as 65%. Neuron protection stems from coffee's caffeine plus its high content of chlorogenic acid and beneficial polyphenols. More significantly, previous studies have shown that coffee helps in the prevention of the two major factors in Alzheimer's development: amyloid plaques and neurofibrillary tangles. Moreover, both caffeine and polyphenols have anti-oxidant effects in reducing inflammation and protecting brain cells in the cortex and hippocampus - the main components responsible for memory.

- Hyberbaric Oxygen Therapy (HBOT) - HBOT is an excellent treatment not only for traumatic and non-traumatic brain injuries but also a host other problems, including infected wounds and circulatory disorders. Many of these situations are precursors of the onset of AD. HBOT involves breathing 100 per cent oxygen in a specialized chamber. This provides an influx of oxygen that sparks energy production and repairs neurons and neuronal connections. The reason HBOT is highlighted here is because approximately 1.5 million Americans visit emergency rooms each year with acute traumatic brain injuries. These injuries are sustained in falls, motor vehicle accidents, assaults and other traumatic incidents. Even though many people recover and regain functions, many do not or even suffer mild repetitive injuries which lead to neurological impairment and the onset of Alzheimer's disease.

Section 4

Weekly Exercise Program

In the fight against the development of Alzheimer's disease, a Weekly Exercise Program is listed below for all persons under 60 with mild cognitive impairment and all persons 60 and over with little or no cognitive impairment.

Monday, Wednesday and Saturday

- Pilates Workout

- Aerobic Exercise

- Brain Aerobics

- Mind-Set Meditation (20 minutes in morning & afternoon)'

Tuesday and Thursday

- Pilates Workout

- Weight Resistant Exercises

- Brain Aerobics

- Mind-Set Meditation

Friday and Sunday
-	Days of Rest from Aerobics

-	Mind-Set Meditation

Every day the following apply:
-	Take vitamin supplements Turmeric and Ubiquinol.

-	Drink 3 - 5 cups of caffeinated coffee.

•	Mind-Set Meditation is optional if you can substitute an alternative process which is effective in removing stress, anxiety and depression.

After much analysis, the author formulated the Weekly Exercise Program in order to give the individual a unique holistic application. This represents a combination of strategies and measures to insure a significant deterrence to onset AD and to provide a minimum group of exercises to insure active life longevity. Looking at all of the material that has been published about AD, no agency has designed or offered a dynamic, comprehensive program of this nature.

To facilitate the exercises, the author has furnished a Pilates Workout sheet which he has custom designed in his capacity as a certified Pilates instructor. Moreover, as a certified Mind-Set Meditation instructor, he has published a book entitled: "Meditation and Spiritual Contemplation" which can be ordered from the author. The author also provides private instruction on this technique. The author originally received the meditation technique from Maharishi Mahesh Yogi in the

French Alps in 1973. In his masters work at USC, his master's thesis on Meditation contained a 40 page narrative and 22 pages of charts.

The Pilates workout is attached. Pilates is a core strengthening exercise which provides greater balance, improved endurance and increased stamina. Performing this exercise at least five times a week will significantly deter joint arthritis.

Pilates Workout

(GREAT FOR BALANCE, ENDURANCE & STAMINA)

DO 10 REPETITIONS (REPS) UNLESS OTHERWISE NOTED

1. ROLL DOWN - Stand erect with arms at your side and slowly reach down (for a six count) to your toes and slowly roll back to an erect standing position.

2. SHOULDER BRIDGE - Lie on back with knees bent. Lift back and pelvis up to form a bridge. Hold for a 6 count.

3. HIP FLEXOR LEG LIFT - Sit-up with legs on floor. Float one leg up & down. Then, do the other. Pelvis remains stationary. Do 30 reps.

4. HEAD PULL-UP - Lie on back with knees bent up with fingers on back of head or on chest. Raise head up & down 4 times. Do 8 reps.

5. LEG-CIRCLE LIFT - Lie on back with one knee bent. Raise leg on floor up in circle and do four fairly wide circles. Then, do the other leg. Pelvis remains stationary.

6.   LEG CROSSOVER - Lie on back with legs on floor. With upper body staying flat on floor, cross one leg over body to far side. Then, do the other leg. Hold for a 6 count.

7.   LEG LIFT/ARM BOUNCE - Lie on back with legs lifted up and bent. Life head. Bounce arms up & down. Do 50 reps.

8.   SCISSOR LEGS - Lie on back. Float legs up. Life head. Scissor legs up & down.

9.   LEG SIDE LIFT - Lie on side with head on arm. Lift leg up and down. Then, turn on the other side and repeat exercise.

10.   SINGLE LEG STAND/ROTATING ARMS -Stand on one leg with other leg back. Bend arms to horizomal position and rotate 10 times from waist out and back. Then, stand on the other leg and repeat arm rotations. Do 5 reps.

11.   SINGLE LEG SQUAT - Stand erect and lunge one leg forward while squatting on the other leg. Alternate leg positions.

12.   ANKLE TO BUTTOCK - Stand erect with hand on ankle of raised leg. Lift ankle to buttock & bend raised knee backwards. Hold for a 50 count.

13.   CALF STRETCH - Lean against a wall with one leg bent forward and the other stretched back making the calf taut. Hold for a 50 count.

14.   CALF RAISE - Stand erect on toes on curb or stair. Lower and raise body. Hold raised position for a 6 count.

15. ROLL DOWN - Stand erect with arms at your side and slowly reach down. (for a six count) to your toes and slowly roll back to an erect standing position.

This workout can be done daily as well as before workouts or major exercises.

Section 5

Summary

The impact of Alzheimer's disease is overwhelming. Looking to the future, the growing numbers of people aging beyond 65 in the United States has the potential to exponentially expand the number of Alzheimer's disease cases well beyond 10 million in the next 10 years.

The only hope in reducing the number of new AD cases other than a cure for AD, is a highly energized and dedicated individual effort. By regularly using the Weekly Exercise Program, the individual is participating in a huge breakthrough which provides a pair of major longevity achievements in mental sharpness and physical health.

NOTE the following pages contain:

1. Meditation And Contemplation summary.

2. A summary of author publications.

Meditation and Spiritual Contemplation

By
TERENCE MCCARTHY

This is an extraordinary primer for meditation and spiritual contemplation (a form of meditation). Meditation is an extremely powerful process which can result in major reduction of SAD - stress, anxiety and depression. SAD can accelerate the development of onset Alzheimers disease.

In addition, studies have shown that the benefits are multi-dimensional. Major improvements have been recorded in the following areas: emotional, mental, physical and spiritual. The unique bottom line is that the meditation process requires no effort or special talent. If one strictly follows the process guidelines, the process works in spite of oneself. Of singular importance is that the person participating in the program must devote two twenty-minute sessions each day to meditating. He leaves the self behind and completely divorces himself from worries, distractions and the material world. The goal is to reach a level of consciousness where there is absolutely nothing. This is otherwise known as a higher state of consciousness which is normally accompanied by a deep state of rest. Every meditator is quite unique. There is no set standard for what a person will or will not experience. The book deals with initial problems of interference and how they are to be handled.

All in all, when one looks at the many significant potential benefits, it can easily be said: if the meditation process were to be participated on a widespread basis across the globe, the changes in world conflict would be reduced considerably and people would be living longer and healthier lives.

This process is not another "la la land" voyage. Terence McCarthy in his introduction offers the following analogy which applies across the board: "Life can be impossibly demanding. There are so many pies that we have our fingers in. Too often, we find that our achievements fall far short f our expectations. This can result in a scattered life style with huge fragmentation. Computers also run into wide-spread scattered situation which require time-consuming searches on a frequent basis. To take care of chis situation, we run a program called "defragmentation". A similar situation develops in our own hectic life styles. The "defragmentation" program chat we need to run is called "meditation".

For Runners over 45: **"RUNNING UNTIL YOU ARE 100"**

This book is the most comprehensive, single source document available that can help you effectively achieve running longevity. Don't miss the opportunity to run into your 90's and lOO's. The author has 43 years of running experience. At 81, he is still active in 8K and 5 K races. In 2015, he entered 63 races and won his age group in 57 events.

For Non-runners over 45: **"ENJOYING LIFE AFTER 55 BY DOING THE RIGHT STUFF"**

This book is a very comprehensive, single source document available to help walkers, cyclists, swimmers, skiers and others to establish a personal program to effectively achieve aerobic exercise longevity.

Don't miss this opportunity to guarantee that you will continue to enjoy your independent life style into your 90's and lOO's.

"MEDITATION AND SPIRITUAL CONTEMPLATION"

Meditation is an extremely powerful process which can result in peace of mind, significant stress reduction and the lowering of blood pressure. Studies have shown major health benefits in the following areas: emotional, mental, physical and spiritual. The author has been meditating for over 40 years. The author provides instruction in this technique.

"FIGHTING ALZHEIMERS DISEASE"

This is easily the most comprehensive book on an exploding health crisis in which everyone over 60 needs to become engaged in a pro-active active program. The strategies and weekly program enumerated will enable an individual co significantly deter the onset of Alzheimers Disease (AD). Of note, 5.3 million Americans have AD. The probability of contracting AD is 13% for people over 65 and 50% over the age of 85.

"POETRY WITH FEELING"

This is a book of 50 rhymed Shakersperian sonnets about various life experiences.

All of the above books can be ordered from amazon.com. Look under the name: "Terence McCarthy".

www.ingramcontent.com/pod-product-compliance
Lightning Source LLC
Chambersburg PA
CBHW070032030426
42335CB00017B/2403